COMPLETE GOUT DIET
COOKBOOK

Quick and Easy Delicious Recipes to Reduce Uric Acid and Conquer Gout Attacks with 14-Day Meal Plan and Quick Tips for Gout Prevention

Dr. Sally J. Keane

TABLE OF CONTENTS

Introduction

Welcome to "A Gout Diet Cookbook," a cookbook designed to transform your connection with food and provide you with the tools you need to manage your gout and improve your general health. This cookbook is a guide for enjoying delectable meals while adhering to the ideals of a gout-friendly lifestyle, not merely a compilation of recipes.

We take you on a culinary journey through the pages that follow, with each dish serving as a tribute to the taste and thoughtful nutrition that work in perfect harmony. Often called the "rich man's disease," gout should not keep you from enjoying the foods and company of the table. Rather, it turns into a chance for culinary ingenuity, investigating a variety of components that satiate the body and the spirit.

Setting the scene, the introduction explains the fundamentals of gout, the importance of dietary decisions, and the multimodal strategy required for successful gout care. Turn the pages to discover a symphony of flavors, from filling breakfasts to fulfilling meals and exquisite snacks, all carefully crafted to conform to gout-friendly guidelines.

This cookbook may serve as your go-to source for delicious recipes as well as the information and ideas you need to live a healthy and flavorful life. Cheers to a voyage of colorful, gout-aware recipes that honor the pleasure of mindful eating and improve your general well-being. Savor the tastes, accept the health benefits, and enjoy every second of this fascinating gastronomic journey.

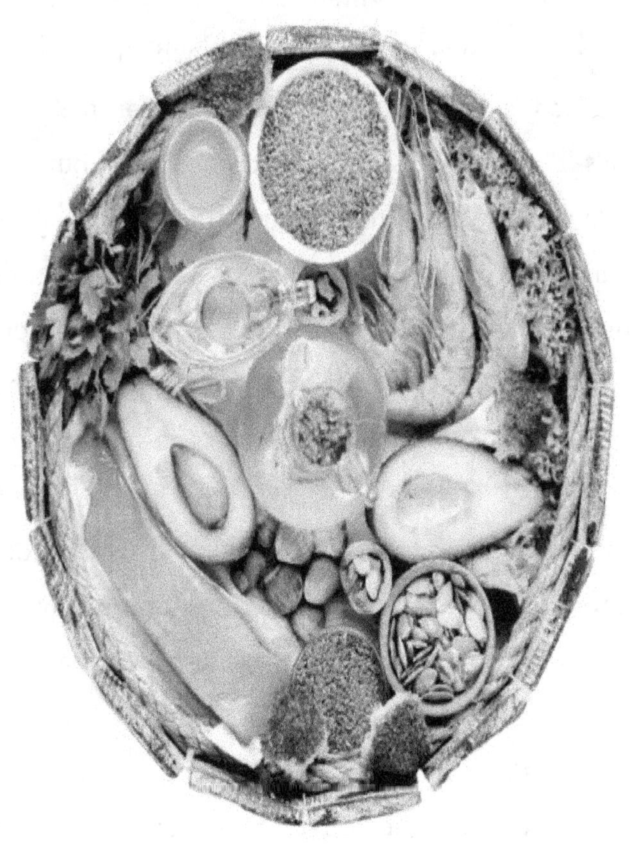

Basics of Gout

When we set out on our culinary adventure with our Gout diet cookbook, it is essential to understand the basics of gout, a condition that permeates many of the recipes we sample. Gout, which is often described as the "disease of kings" or the "rich man's disease," has historical overtones but also exists as a modern problem that affects people from a variety of backgrounds. Here, we break down the fundamentals of gout and create the foundation for a cookbook that is not only aesthetically pleasing but also carefully considered in terms of joint health.

Comprehending Uric Acid Dynamics: Uric acid, a byproduct produced during the digestion of purines present in certain meals and tissues, is essential to the gout process. This cookbook carefully considers the effects of our food selections on uric acid levels as it navigates the culinary environment. The delicate balance between the production and removal of uric acid becomes essential when creating meals that follow gout-friendly guidelines.

Triggers & Culinary Sensitivity: We explore the food triggers that might either exacerbate or lessen gout symptoms in these culinary sections. Purine-rich ingredients like organ meats and red meat play subtle roles in our recipes. Concurrently, our culinary story acknowledges the effect of alcohol and the need of staying hydrated, both of which are critical for managing gout.

Recipes that Reflect Symptoms: This cookbook recognizes the intense pain, swelling, and redness that come with flare-ups as the symptomatic language of gout. Every dish is created with an awareness of the ways in which ingredients may improve joint health in addition to taste. By integrating culinary knowledge with the subtleties of gout symptoms, we provide a setting where each meal serves as a chance to nourish and promote overall wellbeing.

Diagnostic Insights and Lifestyle Synergy: As we taste various tastes, we acknowledge the significance of medical knowledge, lifestyle synergies, and diagnostic insights in the treatment of gout. This cookbook is more than simply a list of recipes; it's a comprehensive resource that combines creative cooking with health-conscious selections, providing a map for anybody attempting to navigate the maze that is gout.

Culinary Considerations Outside the Plate: This cookbook promotes a gout-friendly way of living outside the kitchen. It's a companion that highlights the need of eating well, staying hydrated, and getting regular, fun activity to support joint health. Every dish turns into a chapter in a bigger story, a voyage towards health and deliciousness.

The Role of Diet in Gout Management

The frequency and intensity of gout flare-ups may be greatly influenced by dietary choices, making food a crucial part in managing gout. The hallmark of gout is the buildup of uric acid crystals in the joints, which often causes acute, severe pain. This is a thorough summary of how nutrition affects gout management:

1. **Purine-Rich Foods:** Red meat, organ meats, shellfish, and certain fish varieties are examples of foods strong in purines that might raise uric acid levels. Reducing the amount of these foods consumed decreases the risk of gout attacks and helps to limit the formation of uric acid.

2. **Fructose and Sugary Foods:** Consuming a lot of fructose, which is included in processed foods and sugary drinks, raises uric acid levels and increases the risk of gout. For those who are controlling gout,

consuming sugar-filled meals and drinks in moderation is advised.

3. Alcohol Intake: Because alcohol, especially beer and spirits, contains purines and raises uric acid levels, it may increase an individual's risk of developing gout. It is advised to drink alcohol in moderation or not at all while managing gout.

4. Hydration: Maintaining proper hydration is crucial for managing gout. Getting lots of water into your system facilitates the kidneys' removal of uric acid by diluting it in the blood. The chance of gout flare-ups may be decreased by drinking enough water.

5. Low-Purine Alternatives: The cornerstone of a gout-friendly diet is a focus on foods low in purines, such as fruits, vegetables, whole grains, and low-fat dairy products. These meals promote general health and wellbeing in addition to offering vital nutrients.

6. **Balanced Diet:** Eating a diverse range of nutrient-dense meals guarantees a balanced diet that provides enough nourishment while lowering the risk of gout attacks. Including complex carbs, lean proteins, and healthy fats improves general health and may help control gout symptoms.

7. **Weight Control:** Retaining a healthy weight is essential to managing gout. Being overweight raises the likelihood of gout flare-ups and raises uric acid levels. Maintaining a balanced diet and doing regular exercise help with weight loss and improve joint health.

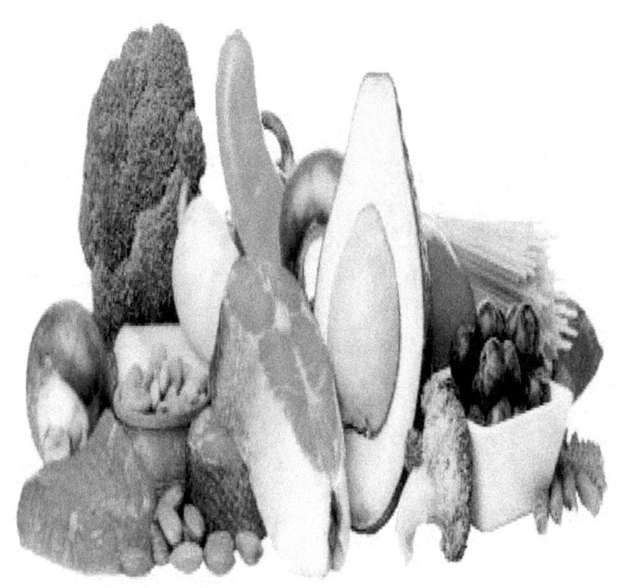

Gout-Friendly Recipes

Recipes that are suitable for those with gout are carefully chosen to conform to dietary guidelines that assist those who are managing the ailment, which is marked by high uric acid levels that cause inflammation in the joints. By using components that are known to have a reduced purine content, these recipes reduce the possibility of inciting gout episodes. Purine-dense red meats and organ meats are often given less importance than lean proteins like fish, chicken, and plant-based substitutes.

The dishes emphasize a lot of fruits and vegetables, which provide anti-inflammatory qualities and important vitamins, minerals, and antioxidants. Whole grains, including brown rice and quinoa, are included to assist weight control and general health, two important facets of gout treatment. Whole grains also contain fiber and complex carbs.

Drinks are also carefully chosen, with water, herbal teas, and other low-calorie, non-sugary alternatives being preferred. Since alcohol is known to raise uric acid levels, it is either avoided or replaced with gout-friendly foods.

Recognizing that excessive calorie intake and abrupt weight fluctuations might affect gout symptoms, portion management is discreetly included. These recipes promote moderation and balance, enabling people to enjoy a wide variety of tastes without jeopardizing their joint health.

In the end, gout-friendly meals provide an experience that goes beyond limitations by emphasizing the colorful and diverse range of components that support general health. Adopting these recipes will allow gout sufferers to enjoy meals that actively support their continued path toward joint health and gout treatment, while also pleasing the palate.

Chapter 1: Breakfast

1. Energizing Quinoa Porridge

INGREDIENTS:

- 1 cup quinoa

- 2 cups almond milk

- 1 tablespoon honey

- 1/2 teaspoon vanilla extract

- 1/4 cup sliced almonds

- Fresh berries for topping

INSTRUCTIONS:

1. Rinse quinoa under cold water.
2. In a saucepan, combine quinoa, almond milk, honey, and vanilla extract.
3. Bring to a boil, then reduce heat and simmer for 15-20 minutes until quinoa is cooked.
4. Serve hot, topped with sliced almonds and fresh berries.

Nutrition per Serving:

- Calories: 350

- Protein: 12g

- Carbohydrates: 55g

- Fat: 9g

- Fiber: 7g

2. Berry Burst Smoothie Bowl

Ingredients:

- 1 cup mixed berries (strawberries, blueberries, raspberries)
- 1 frozen banana
- 1/2 cup Greek yogurt
- 1/4 cup almond milk
- 1 tablespoon chia seeds
- Granola for topping

INSTRUCTIONS:

1. Blend mixed berries, frozen banana, Greek yogurt, and almond milk until smooth.
2. Pour into a bowl and top with chia seeds and granola.

- Calories: 280

- Protein: 10g

- Carbohydrates: 45g

- Fat: 8g

- Fiber: 10g

3. Avocado Toast with Poached Eggs

INGREDIENTS:

- 2 slices whole-grain bread

- 1 ripe avocado

- 2 eggs

- Salt and pepper to taste

- (Optional) red pepper flakes

INSTRUCTIONS:

1. Toast the whole-grain bread slices.

2. Mash ripe avocado and spread it evenly on the toast.

3. Poach eggs and place them on top of the avocado.

4. Carefully season with salt, pepper, and red
    pepper flakes if desired.

Nutrition per Serving:

- Calories: 320

- Protein: 14g

- Carbohydrates: 25g

- Fat: 20g

- Fiber: 8g

4. Spinach and Feta Omelette

INGREDIENTS:

- 3 eggs

- 1/2 cup fresh spinach, chopped

- 2 tablespoons feta cheese, crumbled

- Salt and pepper to taste

- A good cooking spray or olive oil for the pan

INSTRUCTIONS:

1. Whisk eggs in a bowl and season with salt
    and pepper very well

2. Heat a pan, add cooking spray or olive oil.

3. Pour whisked eggs into the pan, add chopped spinach and feta.

4. Cook until the omelette sets, then fold and serve.

Nutrition per Serving:

- Calories: 280

- Protein: 20g

- Carbohydrates: 3g

- Fat: 20g

- Fiber: 2g

5. Greek Yogurt Parfait with Nuts

INGREDIENTS:

- 1 cup Greek yogurt

- 1/2 cup granola

- 1/4 cup mixed nuts (almonds, walnuts, pistachios)

- 1 tablespoon honey

- Fresh berries for topping

INSTRUCTIONS:

1. Layer Greek yogurt, granola, and mixed nuts in a glass or bowl.
2. Drizzle honey on top and add fresh berries.

Nutrition per Serving:

- Calories: 350

- Protein: 18g

- Carbohydrates: 30g

- Fat: 18g

- Fiber: 5g

6.   Blueberry   Buckwheat Pancakes

INGREDIENTS:

- 1 cup buckwheat flour

- 1 teaspoon baking powder

- 1/2 teaspoon cinnamon

- 1 cup almond milk

- 1 egg

- 1 cup fresh blueberries

- Maple syrup for drizzling

INSTRUCTIONS:

1. In a bowl, mix buckwheat flour, baking powder, and cinnamon.
2. Add almond milk and egg, stir until well combined.
3. Gently fold in fresh blueberries.
4. Cook pancakes well on a griddle until golden brown on both sides.
5. Serve with a drizzle of maple syrup.

Nutrition per Serving:

- Calories: 280
- Protein: 9g
- Carbohydrates: 50g
- Fat: 5g
- Fiber: 8g

7. Chia Seed Pudding with Mango

INGREDIENTS:

- 1/4 cup chia seeds
- 1 cup coconut milk
- 1 tablespoon honey

- 1/2 teaspoon vanilla extract

- Fresh mango slices for topping

INSTRUCTIONS:

1. Mix chia seeds, coconut milk, honey, and vanilla extract in a bowl.

2. Refrigerate for at least four hours or overnight, allowing the chia seeds to absorb the liquid very well.

3. Stir well before serving and top with fresh mango slices.

Nutrition per Serving:

- Calories: 220

- Protein: 5g

- Carbohydrates: 25g

- Fat: 12g

- Fiber: 10g

8. Sweet Potato and Turkey Breakfast Hash

INGREDIENTS:

- 1 sweet potato, diced
- 1/2 pound ground turkey
- 1 bell pepper, chopped
- 1 onion, diced
- 1 teaspoon smoked paprika
- Salt and pepper to taste
- Fresh parsley for garnish

INSTRUCTIONS:

1. In a skillet, brown ground turkey.
2. Add diced sweet potato, bell pepper, and onion. Cook until vegetables are tender.
3. Season with smoked paprika, salt, and pepper.
4. Garnish with fresh parsley before serving.

Nutrition per Serving:

- Calories: 320
- Protein: 18g

- Carbohydrates: 30g

- Fat: 15g

- Fiber: 6g

9. Whole Grain Waffles with Berries

INGREDIENTS:

- 1 cup whole wheat flour

- 1 tablespoon baking powder

- 1 tablespoon honey

- 1 cup almond milk

- 1 egg

- Mixed berries for topping

- Greek yogurt for serving

INSTRUCTIONS:

1. Mix whole wheat flour, baking powder, honey, almond milk, and egg in a bowl.

2. Pour batter into a waffle maker and cook until golden.

3. Top with mixed berries and serve with a dollop of Greek yogurt.

- Calories: 250

- Protein: 10g

- Carbohydrates: 40g

- Fat: 5g

- Fiber: 7g

10. Egg and Veggie Muffins

INGREDIENTS:

- 6 eggs

- 1/2 cup diced bell peppers

- 1/2 cup chopped spinach

- 1/4 cup feta cheese, crumbled

- Salt and pepper to taste

INSTRUCTIONS:

1. Preheat the oven to 350°F (175°C).

2. Whisk eggs and season with salt and pepper.

3. Stir in diced bell peppers, chopped spinach, and crumbled feta.

4. Pour the mixture into muffin cups and bake for 15-20 minutes until set.

Nutrition per Serving:
- Calories: 180
- Protein: 12g
- Carbohydrates: 3g
- Fat: 14g
- Fiber: 1g

Chapter 2: Lunch

11. Grilled Salmon Salad with Citrus Vinaigrette

INGREDIENTS:

- 2 salmon fillets

- Mixed salad greens

- Cherry tomatoes, halved

- Cucumber, sliced

- 1 orange, segmented

- 2 tablespoons olive oil

- 1 tablespoon balsamic vinegar

- Salt and pepper to taste

INSTRUCTIONS:

1. Season salmon fillets with salt and pepper, grill until cooked.

2. Arrange mixed salad greens, cherry tomatoes, cucumber, and orange segments on a plate.

3. Place grilled salmon on top.

4. Whisk together olive oil and balsamic vinegar for the vinaigrette, drizzle over the salad.

Nutrition per Serving:

- Calories: 400

- Protein: 30g

- Carbohydrates: 15g

- Fat: 25g

- Fiber: 5g

12. Quinoa and Chickpea Buddha Bowl

INGREDIENTS:

- 1 cup cooked quinoa
- 1 cup chickpeas, drained and rinsed
- Mixed vegetables (e.g., broccoli, carrots, bell peppers)
- 2 tablespoons tahini
- Lemon juice
- Salt and pepper to taste

INSTRUCTIONS:

1. Roast chickpeas and mixed vegetables in the oven.

2. Assemble a bowl with cooked quinoa, roasted chickpeas, and vegetables.

3. Drizzle with tahini and lemon juice, season with salt and pepper.

Nutrition per Serving:

- Calories: 380
- Protein: 15g
- Carbohydrates: 55g
- Fat: 12g
- Fiber: 10g

13. Turkey and Veggie Wrap with Hummus

INGREDIENTS:

- Whole-grain tortilla
- 1/2 cup cooked ground turkey
- Hummus
- Mixed greens
- Cherry tomatoes, sliced

- Red onion, thinly sliced

INSTRUCTIONS:

1. Spread hummus on a whole-grain tortilla.
2. Add cooked ground turkey, mixed greens, cherry tomatoes, and red onion.
3. Gently roll into a wrap and slice in half.

Nutrition per Serving:

- Calories: 320
- Protein: 20g
- Carbohydrates: 30g
- Fat: 15g
- Fiber: 8g

14. Lentil Soup with Spinach and Tomatoes

INGREDIENTS:

- 1 cup dried lentils
- 1 onion, chopped
- 2 carrots, diced
- 2 tomatoes, diced
- 3 cups vegetable broth

- 2 cups fresh spinach

- 1 teaspoon cumin

- Salt and pepper to taste

INSTRUCTIONS:

1. Rinse lentils and combine with chopped onion, carrots, tomatoes, and vegetable broth in a pot.
2. Simmer until lentils are tender.
3. Add fresh spinach, cumin, salt, and pepper. Cook until spinach wilts.

Nutrition per Serving:

- Calories: 250

- Protein: 18g

- Carbohydrates: 40g

- Fat: 2g

- Fiber: 15g

15. Mediterranean Chicken Skewers

INGREDIENTS:

- One pound chicken breast, cut into cubes

- Cherry tomatoes

- Red onion, cut into chunks

- Bell peppers, cut into chunks

- Olive oil

- Lemon juice

- Garlic, minced

- Oregano, dried

- Salt and pepper to taste

INSTRUCTIONS:

1. In a bowl, mix chicken, cherry tomatoes, red onion, and bell peppers.

2. In a separate bowl, whisk together olive oil, lemon juice, minced garlic, dried oregano, salt, and pepper.

3. Marinate chicken and vegetables in the mixture for at least 30 minutes.

4. Skewer the marinated ingredients and grill
    until chicken is cooked.

Nutrition per Serving:

- Calories: 280

- Protein: 30g

- Carbohydrates: 10g

- Fat: 12g

- Fiber: 3g

16. Shrimp and Quinoa Stuffed Peppers

INGREDIENTS:

- 4 bell peppers, halved

- 1 cup cooked quinoa

- 1/2 pound shrimp, gently peeled and deveined

- Cherry tomatoes, halved

- 1 cup spinach, chopped

- Feta cheese, crumbled

- Olive oil

- Lemon zest

- Salt and pepper to taste

INSTRUCTIONS:

1. Preheat the oven to 375°F (190°C).

2. In a pan, cook shrimp in olive oil until pink.

3. Combine cooked quinoa, shrimp, cherry tomatoes, spinach, feta, lemon zest, salt, and pepper.

4. Carefully stuff bell peppers with the mixture and bake until peppers are tender.

Nutrition per Serving:

- Calories: 320
- Protein: 25g
- Carbohydrates: 30g
- Fat: 12g
- Fiber: 7g

17. Caprese Salad with Balsamic Glaze

INGREDIENTS:

- Tomatoes, sliced
- Fresh mozzarella cheese, sliced
- Fresh basil leaves
- Balsamic glaze

- Olive oil

- Salt and pepper to taste

INSTRUCTIONS:

1. Arrange tomato and mozzarella slices gently
    on a plate or dish.
2. Tuck fresh basil leaves between the slices.
3. Drizzle with balsamic glaze and olive oil.
4. Season with salt and pepper.

Nutrition per Serving:

- Calories: 250

- Protein: 12g

- Carbohydrates: 5g

- Fat: 20g

- Fiber: 1g

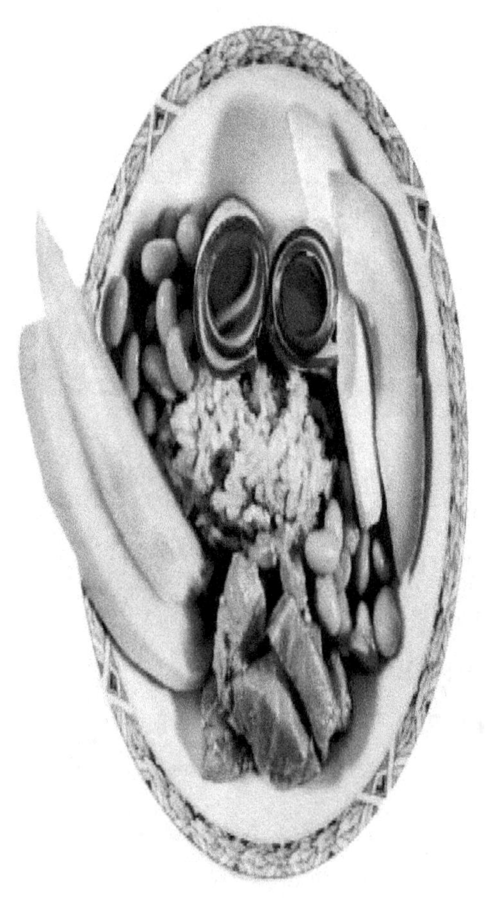

Chapter 3: Dinner Delicacies

18. Baked Cod with Lemon and Herbs

INGREDIENTS:

- 4 cod fillets

- Lemon zest

- Fresh thyme

- Garlic, minced

- Olive oil

- Salt and pepper to taste

INSTRUCTIONS:

1. Preheat the oven to 400°F (200°C).

2. Place cod fillets on a baking sheet.

3. Mix lemon zest, fresh thyme, minced garlic, olive oil, salt, and pepper.

4. Brush the mixture over the cod fillets.

5. Bake for fifteen-twenty minutes or until the fish flakes easily.

<u>*Nutrition per Serving:*</u>

- Calories: 200

- Protein: 25g

- Carbohydrates: 2g

- Fat: 10g, Fiber: 1g

19. Cauliflower Rice Stir-Fry with Tofu

INGREDIENTS:

- 1 head cauliflower, riced

- 1 block firm tofu, cubed

- Mixed vegetables (broccoli, bell peppers, carrots)

- Soy sauce

- Sesame oil

- Ginger, grated

- Garlic, minced

- Green onions for garnish

INSTRUCTIONS:

1. Stir-fry tofu until golden in sesame oil.

2. Add mixed vegetables, grated ginger, and minced garlic.

3. Stir in cauliflower rice and soy sauce.

4. Cook until vegetables are tender.

5. Garnish with chopped green onions.

Nutrition per Serving:

- Calories: 280, Protein: 18g

- Carbohydrates: 20g

- Fat: 15g, Fiber: 8g

20. Zucchini Noodles with Pesto and Cherry Tomatoes

INGREDIENTS:

- Zucchini, spiralized into noodles

- Cherry tomatoes, halved

- Pesto sauce

- Pine nuts

- Parmesan cheese, grated

- Salt and pepper to taste

INSTRUCTIONS:

1. Sauté zucchini noodles until tender.

2. Toss with cherry tomatoes, pesto sauce, and pine nuts.

3. Season with salt and pepper.

4. Sprinkle with grated Parmesan cheese before serving.

Nutrition per Serving:

- Calories: 220

- Protein: 8g

- Carbohydrates: 15g

- Fat: 15g

- Fiber: 5g

21. Beef and Vegetable Kebabs

INGREDIENTS:

- 1 pound lean beef, cubed

- Bell peppers, onions, cherry tomatoes for skewering

- Olive oil

- Garlic powder

- Paprika

- Cumin

- Salt and pepper to taste

INSTRUCTIONS:

1. Preheat the grill.

2. Thread beef and vegetables onto skewers.

3. Brush with olive oil and sprinkle with garlic powder, paprika, cumin, salt, and pepper.

4. Grill very well until beef is cooked to your liking.

<u>Nutrition per Serving:</u>

- Calories: 300

- Protein: 25g

- Carbohydrates: 10g

- Fat: 18g

- Fiber: 3g

22. Stuffed Bell Peppers with Quinoa and Black Beans

INGREDIENTS:

- Bell peppers, halved

- 1 cup cooked quinoa

- One cup black beans, well drained and rinsed

- Corn kernels

- Salsa

- Mexican cheese blend

- Cilantro for garnish

INSTRUCTIONS:

1. Preheat the oven to 375°F (190°C).

2. Mix cooked quinoa, black beans, corn, and salsa together.

3. Stuff bell peppers with the quinoa mixture.

4. Top with Mexican cheese blend.

5. Bake until peppers are tender.

6. Garnish with chopped cilantro.

Nutrition per Serving:

- Calories: 320

- Protein: 15g

- Carbohydrates: 45g

- Fat: 8g

- Fiber: 12g

23. Lemon Garlic Chicken with Asparagus

INGREDIENTS:

- 4 boneless, skinless chicken breasts

- Asparagus spears

- Lemon juice

- Garlic, minced

- Olive oil

- Fresh parsley, chopped

- Salt and pepper to taste

INSTRUCTIONS:

1. Preheat the oven to 400°F (200°C).

2. Season chicken breasts with salt, pepper, and minced garlic.

3. Place chicken on a baking sheet with asparagus spears.

4. Drizzle with olive oil and lemon juice.

5. Bake until the chicken is cooked through and asparagus is tender.

6. Garnish with chopped fresh parsley.

<u>***Nutrition per Serving:***</u>

- Calories: 280

- Protein: 30g

- Carbohydrates: 8g

- Fat: 12g

- Fiber: 3g

24. Eggplant and Chickpea Curry

INGREDIENTS:

- 1 large eggplant, diced

- One can chickpeas, well drained and rinsed

- Onion, chopped

- Garlic, minced

- Ginger, grated

- Curry powder

- Coconut milk

- Cilantro for garnish

- Basmati rice for serving

INSTRUCTIONS:

1. In a pan, sauté chopped onion, minced garlic, and grated ginger.
2. Add diced eggplant and chickpeas, cook until eggplant is tender.
3. Stir in curry powder and coconut milk.
4. Simmer until the curry thickens.
5. Garnish with chopped cilantro and serve over basmati rice.

Nutrition per Serving:

- Calories: 320
- Protein: 10g
- Carbohydrates: 40g
- Fat: 15g
- Fiber: 12g

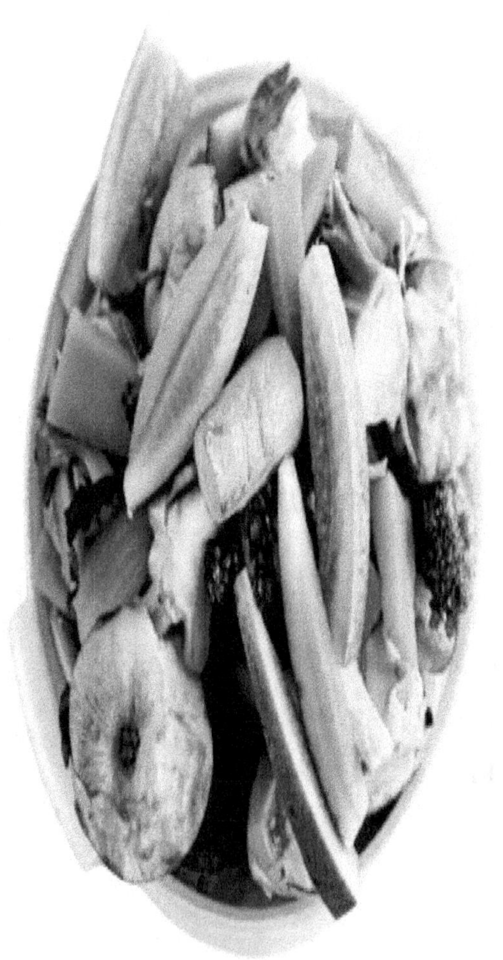

Chapter 4: Snacks and Desserts

25. Guacamole with Veggie Sticks

INGREDIENTS:

- 2 ripe avocados

- 1 tomato, diced

- 1/4 cup of red onion, well and finely chopped

- 1 clove garlic, minced

- Lime juice

- Salt and pepper to taste

- Carrot and cucumber fruit sticks for dipping

INSTRUCTIONS:

1. Mash avocados in a bowl.

2. Stir in diced tomato, chopped red onion, minced garlic, and lime juice.

3. Season with salt and pepper.

4. Serve with carrot and cucumber sticks.

- Calories: 150

- Protein: 2g

- Carbohydrates: 10g

- Fat: 12g

- Fiber: 6g

26. Roasted Chickpeas with Turmeric

INGREDIENTS:

- One can chickpeas, well drained and rinsed

- Olive oil

- Turmeric powder

- Cumin

- Paprika

- Salt and pepper to taste

INSTRUCTIONS:

1. Preheat the oven to 400°F (200°C).

2. Toss chickpeas with olive oil, turmeric, cumin, paprika, salt, and pepper.

3. Spread chickpeas on a baking sheet.

4. Roast until crispy, stirring occasionally.

- Calories: 120

- Protein: 5g

- Carbohydrates: 15g

- Fat: 4g

- Fiber: 5g

27. Greek Yogurt Dip with Cucumber Slices

INGREDIENTS:

- 1 cup Greek yogurt

- 1/2 cucumber, diced

- Fresh dill, chopped

- Lemon zest

- Salt and pepper to taste

INSTRUCTIONS:

1. Mix Greek yogurt with diced cucumber, chopped fresh dill, and lemon zest.

2. Season with salt and pepper.

3. Chill before serving with cucumber slices.

<u>***Nutrition per Serving:***</u>

- Calories: 90

- Protein: 10g

- Carbohydrates: 6g

- Fat: 3g

- Fiber: 1g

28. Almond and Berry Trail Mix

INGREDIENTS:

- Almonds

- Dried blueberries

- Dried cranberries

- Dark chocolate chunks

- Coconut flakes

INSTRUCTIONS:

1. Mix almonds, dried blueberries, dried cranberries, dark chocolate chunks, and coconut flakes.

2. Portion into snack-sized bags for convenient munching.

**Nutrition per Serving:**

- Calories: 200

- Protein: 5g

- Carbohydrates: 15g

- Fat: 14g

- Fiber: 4g

29. Hummus-Stuffed Mini Peppers

INGREDIENTS:

- Mini bell peppers

- Hummus

- Cherry tomatoes, halved

- Fresh parsley, chopped

INSTRUCTIONS:

1. Slice mini bell peppers in half.

2. Fill each half with hummus.

3. Top with halved cherry tomatoes and chopped fresh parsley.

*<u>**Nutrition per Serving:**</u>*

- Calories: 120

- Protein: 4g

- Carbohydrates: 15g

- Fat: 6g

- Fiber: 4g

30. Avocado and Tomato Salsa

INGREDIENTS:

- 2 avocados, diced

- 1 cup cherry tomatoes, diced

- Red onion, finely chopped

- Fresh cilantro, chopped

- Lime juice

- Salt and pepper to taste

- Whole grain tortilla chips for dipping

INSTRUCTIONS:

1. Combine diced avocados, cherry tomatoes, chopped red onion, and fresh cilantro.

2. Squeeze lime juice over the mixture.

3. Season with salt and pepper.

4. Serve with whole grain tortilla chips.

Nutrition per Serving:

- Calories: 160

- Protein: 2g

- Carbohydrates: 12g

- Fat: 13g

- Fiber: 5g

31. Edamame and Sea Salt

INGREDIENTS:

- Edamame pods

- Sea salt

INSTRUCTIONS:

1. Boil or steam edamame pods until tender.

2. Sprinkle with sea salt.

3. Serve as a healthy and protein-packed snack.

Nutrition per Serving:

- Calories: 90

- Protein: 8g

- Carbohydrates: 8g

- Fat: 3g

- Fiber: 4g

32. Cottage Cheese and Pineapple Cups

INGREDIENTS:

- Cottage cheese

- Fresh pineapple, diced

- Mint leaves for garnish

INSTRUCTIONS:

1. Spoon cottage cheese into individual cups.

2. Top with diced fresh pineapple.

3. Garnish with mint leaves before serving.

Nutrition per Serving:

- Calories: 120

- Protein: 15g

- Carbohydrates: 10g

- Fat: 2g

- Fiber: 1g

33. Spicy Kale Chips

INGREDIENTS:

- Fresh kale, stems removed and torn into pieces

- Olive oil

- Chili powder

- Garlic powder

- Paprika

- Salt

INSTRUCTIONS:

1. Preheat the oven to 350°F (175°C).

2. Massage kale with olive oil, chili powder, garlic powder, paprika, and a pinch of salt.

3. Bake until crisp, about 10-15 minutes.

Nutrition per Serving:

- Calories: 70

- Protein: 3g

- Carbohydrates: 8g

- Fat: 4g

- Fiber: 2g

34. Nut Butter Banana Bites

INGREDIENTS:

- Banana, sliced

- Nut butter either (almond, peanut, or your choice)

- Chia seeds

INSTRUCTIONS:

1. Spread nut butter on banana slices.

2. Sprinkle with chia seeds.

3. Enjoy as a quick and nutritious bite-sized snack.

Nutrition per Serving:

- Calories: 100

- Protein: 3g

- Carbohydrates: 15g

- Fat: 5g

- Fiber: 3g

14-Day Meal Plan for Gout Diet

Day 1:

- **Breakfast:** Energizing Quinoa Porridge
- **Lunch:** Grilled Salmon Salad with Citrus Vinaigrette
- **Dinner:** Baked Cod with Lemon and Herbs
- **Snack:** Guacamole with Veggie Sticks

Day 2:

- **Breakfast:** Berry Burst Smoothie Bowl
- **Lunch:** Quinoa and Chickpea Buddha Bowl
- **Dinner:** Cauliflower Rice Stir-Fry with Tofu
- **Snack:** Roasted Chickpeas with Turmeric

Day 3:

- **Breakfast:** Avocado Toast with Poached Eggs
- **Lunch:** Turkey and Veggie Wrap with Hummus
- **Dinner:** Zucchini Noodles with Pesto and Cherry Tomatoes
- **Snack:** Greek Yogurt Parfait with Nuts

Day 4:

- **Breakfast:** Spinach and Feta Omelette
- **Lunch:** Lentil Soup with Spinach and Tomatoes
- **Dinner:** Beef and Vegetable Kebabs
- **Snack:** Almond and Berry Trail Mix

Day 5:

- **Breakfast:** Blueberry Buckwheat Pancakes
- **Lunch:** Mediterranean Chicken Skewers
- **Dinner:** Stuffed Bell Peppers with Quinoa and Black Beans
- **Snack:** Hummus-Stuffed Mini Peppers

Day 6:

- **Breakfast:** Chia Seed Pudding with Mango
- **Lunch:** Shrimp and Quinoa Stuffed Peppers
- **Dinner:** Lemon Garlic Chicken with Asparagus
- **Snack:** Avocado and Tomato Salsa

Day 7:

- **Breakfast:** Sweet Potato and Turkey Breakfast Hash
- **Lunch:** Caprese Salad with Balsamic Glaze
- **Dinner:** Eggplant and Chickpea Curry
- **Snack:** Edamame and Sea Salt

Day 8:

- **Breakfast:** Whole Grain Waffles with Berries
- **Lunch:** Greek Yogurt Dip with Cucumber Slices
- **Dinner:** Nut Butter Banana Bites
- **Snack:** Cottage Cheese and Pineapple Cups

Day 9:

- **Breakfast:** Egg and Veggie Muffins
- **Lunch:** Quinoa and Chickpea Buddha Bowl
- **Dinner:** Baked Cod with Lemon and Herbs
- **Snack:** Spicy Kale Chips

Day 10:

- **Breakfast:** Berry Burst Smoothie Bowl
- **Lunch:** Grilled Salmon Salad with Citrus Vinaigrette
- **Dinner:** Cauliflower Rice Stir-Fry with Tofu
- **Snack:** Guacamole with Veggie Sticks

Day 11:

- **Breakfast:** Avocado Toast with Poached Eggs
- **Lunch:** Turkey and Veggie Wrap with Hummus
- **Dinner:** Zucchini Noodles with Pesto and Cherry Tomatoes
- **Snack:** Roasted Chickpeas with Turmeric

Day 12:

- **Breakfast:** Spinach and Feta Omelette
- **Lunch:** Lentil Soup with Spinach and Tomatoes
- **Dinner:** Beef and Vegetable Kebabs
- **Snack:** Almond and Berry Trail Mix

Day 13:

- **Breakfast:** Blueberry Buckwheat Pancakes
- **Lunch:** Mediterranean Chicken Skewers
- **Dinner:** Stuffed Bell Peppers with Quinoa and Black Beans
- **Snack:** Hummus-Stuffed Mini Peppers

Day 14:

- **Breakfast:** Chia Seed Pudding with Mango
- **Lunch:** Shrimp and Quinoa Stuffed Peppers
- **Dinner:** Lemon Garlic Chicken with Asparagus
- **Snack:** Avocado and Tomato Salsa

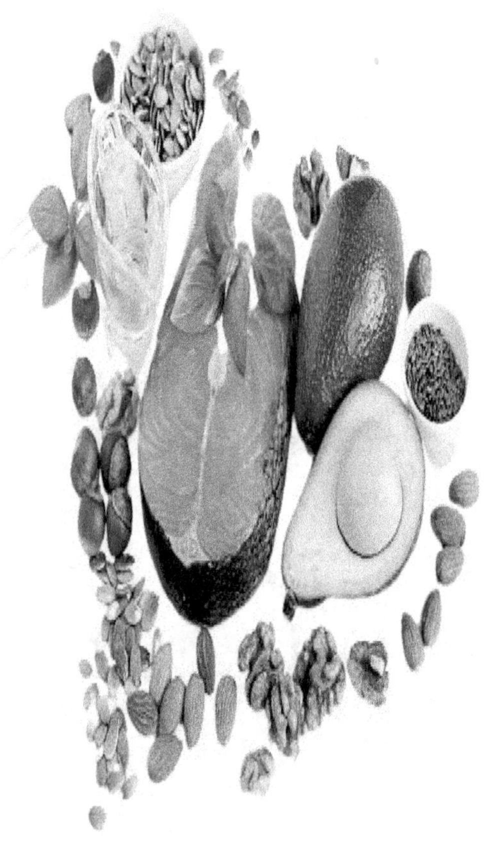

Conclusion

Throughout the pages of this Gout diet cookbook, we stand at the intersection of flavor and well-being, having unraveled the intricate relationship between our culinary choices and the effective management of gout. As we reflect on the lessons learned and the recipes shared, let this conclusion be a melodic ensemble of appreciation, education, and encouragement.

First and foremost, we extend our heartfelt appreciation for embarking on this culinary odyssey. Your dedication to exploring gout-friendly recipes signifies a commitment to your health that deserves commendation. Each recipe you've encountered within these pages is a labor of love, crafted with the intention to tantalize your taste buds while respecting the delicate balance required for gout management.

Throughout our journey, we've delved into the basics of gout, deciphering the language of uric acid, and understanding the triggers that can either spark or soothe gout symptoms. The role of diet in managing gout emerged as a powerful ally, offering strategic choices, embracing lean proteins, and celebrating the abundance of fruits and vegetables. The cookbook has served as both a guide and an educational tool, empowering you to make informed decisions for your joint health.

As you close the final chapter of this cookbook, let it not mark an endpoint but rather a launching pad for sustained well-being. The gout-friendly lifestyle extends beyond these recipes, encompassing daily choices in hydration, exercise, and mindful indulgence. This conclusion is an encouragement to carry the knowledge gained into your everyday life, creating a symphony of health where every ingredient plays a crucial role.

In essence, this cookbook is not just a collection of recipes; it's a culinary symphony composed for your well-being. Each dish resonates with the harmony of flavor and health-conscious choices. It is our hope that as you savor these creations, you find not only delight in every bite but also a pathway to a future where gout management becomes an integral part of your vibrant and fulfilling life.

May every meal be a celebration of good health, and may your culinary adventures continue to unfold with joy, flavor, and a profound commitment to well-being. Thank you for being a part of this transformative journey.

Appendix

Grocery Shopping Guide

Starting a profitable grocery store business is essential to living a gout-friendly lifestyle. The purpose of this book is to provide you with the information and techniques required to make wise decisions when navigating the aisles. Let's explore important factors to take into account for a deliberate and health-conscious grocery shopping experience.

1. Embrace the Perimeter: Take some time to go around the store's perimeter as you begin your supermarket adventure. Fresh fruit, lean meats, dairy products, and whole grains are usually found here. Choosing healthy, fresh foods is the first step toward a cart that is gout-friendly.

2. Select Vibrant Fruits and Vegetables: Stuff your basket with an assortment of vibrant fruits and veggies. These nutrient-dense alternatives enhance your meals with a variety of tastes while also improving your general health. To guarantee a wide range of vitamins and minerals, strive for diversity.

3. Lean Proteins: Pick lean protein sources including beans, fish, chicken, and tofu. Without the increased purine level often seen in red meats, these choices provide vital protein. Adding several types of proteins to your dishes makes them more versatile.

4. healthy Grains and Low-Fat Dairy: Choose low-fat dairy products and load your shopping with healthy grains like quinoa, brown rice, and oats. These options provide fiber, vital minerals, and a well-balanced base for your meals that are suitable for those with gout.

5. Be Mindful of Dairy: Select low-fat or fat-free dairy products when making your choice. For example, yogurt may be a great source of protein and probiotics. To be sure the decisions you're making are in line with your gout treatment objectives, thoroughly read the labels.

6. Choose Wise Snacking Selections: When it comes to snacking, choose gout-friendly selections. Consider fresh fruits with nuts or seeds. Refined sugar and saturated fat snacks should be avoided since they may aggravate flare-ups of gout.

7. Examine Labels to Find Hidden Offenders: Read labels carefully. Elevated uric acid levels may be caused by hidden chemicals found in some packaged meals. Be wary of preservatives, additives, and high sodium levels.

8. Drink Water Sensibly: Water is a gout-friendly remedy. Select water above sugary drinks to stay hydrated. A taste boost without additional sweets may be achieved using herbal teas and infused water.

9. Make a List and Plan Ahead: Based on your meal plan, make a thorough shopping list before you go to the store. This keeps you on task, curbs impulsive buying, and guarantees that you have everything you need for your gout-friendly dishes.

10. While fresh produce is preferable, frozen or canned fruits and vegetables may serve as handy substitutes. Just watch out for salt and extra sugars in canned foods. Choose foods without additional syrups or sauces.

11. Take into Account Gout-Friendly Supplements: If necessary, discuss gout-friendly supplements like vitamin C or cherry extract with your healthcare physician. You may include them into your regimen to get even more help.

12. Stay Seasonal: Selecting seasonal vegetables may save costs while also improving taste. The nutritional content of seasonal fruits and vegetables is often at its highest.

You may turn grocery shopping into an opportunity to promote your gout-friendly lifestyle by embracing these concepts and approaching it mindfully and with a plan. I hope you fill your shopping basket with colorful, healthful options that enhance your overall wellbeing. Happy, mindful-of-your-health shopping!

Quick Tips for Gout Prevention

A combination of food decisions, lifestyle modifications, and mindful practices are used to avoid gout. The following brief advice can assist you in avoiding gout flare-ups and preserving ideal joint health:

1. Drink Plenty of Water: Proper hydration aids in uric acid excretion, which lowers blood uric acid levels. Try to drink 64 ounces or at least 8 glasses of water per day.

2. Adopt a Gout-Friendly Diet: Use lean proteins, whole grains, fruits, and vegetables in a well-balanced diet.
- Restrict your consumption of foods high in purines, such as organ meats, red meat, and certain shellfish.
- Portion control and a variety of meals should be enjoyed in moderation.

3. Select Low-Fat Dairy: Add low-fat dairy products to your diet. Milk and yogurt may be good sources of protein and calcium without raising blood uric acid levels.

4. Limit Alcohol Intake: Since beer and spirits are associated with a higher risk of gout, it is advisable to limit your intake of alcohol. Think of wine as a possible safer alternative when consumed in moderation.

5. Effectively Manage Your Weight: Keep your weight in check by combining a nutritious diet with frequent exercise. Maintaining a healthy weight is essential for avoiding gout.

6. Work Out Frequently: Take up low-impact activities like cycling, swimming, or strolling. Frequent exercise improves joint health, aids in weight management, and may lessen the frequency of gout episodes.

7. Track Your Uric Acid Levels: Regular blood testing to measure your uric acid levels will help you keep tabs on your progress and assist you make dietary and lifestyle improvements.

8. Take Into Account Gout-Friendly Supplements: Talk to your doctor about supplements like vitamin C or cherry extract that may help avoid gout.

9. Mindful Medication Management: Follow your doctor's instructions if you are taking medication to avoid gout. Taking prescription drugs as directed may be an essential part of controlling uric acid levels.

10. Stress Management: Engage in stress-relieving activities like yoga, meditation, or mindfulness. Gout flare-ups may be exacerbated by ongoing stress.

11. Limit Sugar and Processed Foods: Cut less on sugar-filled drinks, processed meals, and fructose-rich foods. These decisions might be a factor in high uric acid levels.

12. Educate Yourself: Learn about the causes and symptoms of gout. Being knowledgeable allows you to take proactive measures to maintain the health of your joints.

Happy Cooking!